SOMATIC EXERCISE FOR TRAUMA RELEASE

A Therapeutic Journey To Calm The Mind Rebalances The Body And Nurture Overall Well-Being.

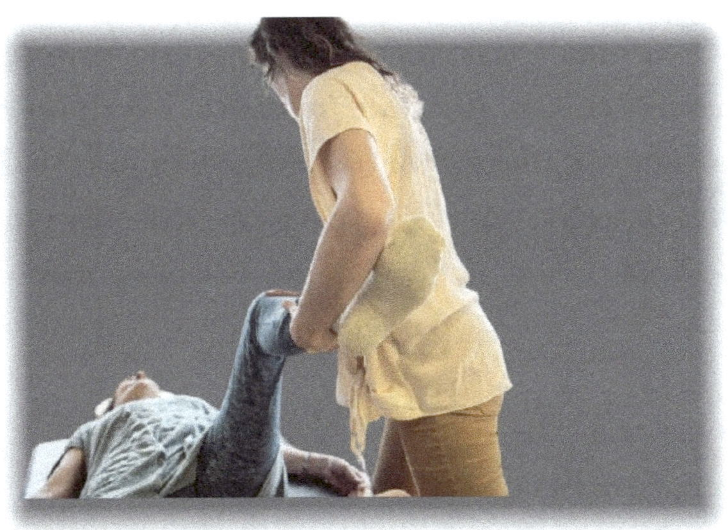

SARAH J. HALLMAN

Copyright Page

© 2024 [SARAH J. HALLMAN]

This book is a work of non-fiction. Names, characters, places, and incidents are either the product of the author's imagination or are used fictitiously. Any resemblance to actual persons, living or dead, events, or locales is entirely coincidental.

Cover design by [**SARAH J. HALLMAN**]

Published by [**SARAH J. HALLMAN**]

OPENING REMARKS

Within the fields of therapeutic methods and holistic wellness, somatic exercises are particularly effective instruments for fostering recovery and wellbeing. Based in the knowledge of the mind-body link, somatic exercises provide a special way to deal with problems related to the physical, mental, and emotional spheres. By use of breath work, conscious movement, and sensory awareness, people set out on a path of self-discovery and metamorphosis, frequently resulting in significant changes in their general health and energy.

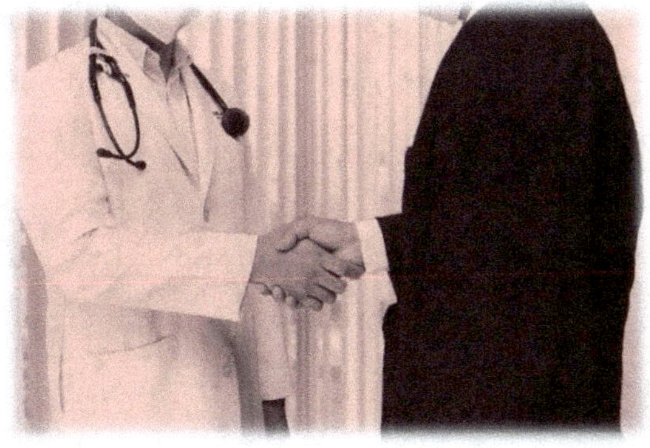

To really understand the powerful effects of somatic exercises, let us tell the tale of John, a middle-aged man who used these techniques to find comfort and healing. John's story is proof positive that somatic exercises can help people recover their sense of self and overcome trauma.

Journey of Scott

Scott had excelled academically all his life. Successful businessman, he flourished in the hectic field of corporate finance. Beneath the surface of achievement, Scott, though, bore a tremendous load that he had been carrying for far too long.

Scott learned to suppress his emotions deep within himself from growing up in a turbulent home characterized by emotional abuse and neglect. The years passed and this emotional repression finally showed out as anxiety, chronic stress, and a sense of alienation from his body.

Though Scott was successful on the outside, he was struggling inside. He battled anxiousness all the time, insomnia, and panic attacks. Although conventional treatment provided some comfort, Scott wanted more—a comprehensive strategy that would deal with the underlying reason of his misery.

Scott initially heard of somatic exercises through a coincidental meeting with a friend. He was drawn to the unusual route to recovery after learning that movement might be used to treat trauma.

Scott started his somatic investigation under the direction of an experienced somatic therapist. He was first dubious about the possibility that anything as basic as conscious movement might relieve years of emotional suffering. But when he gave the practice his whole attention, Scott started to feel significant changes in both his body and mind.

Scott discovered how to re-establish connections with long-forgotten sensations through soft motions and breath work. He found deep-seated muscle knots that he was releasing with every deliberate action. Scott had never imagined a sense of release as he profoundly inhaled into places of pain.

Scott started to relax physically and mentally with every session. He came upon a fresh, present-oriented experience of embodied presence. Scott had been searching for peace in the present moment all his life, but now he was free from the demons of his past.

Weeks went months, and everybody around Scott could see he was changing. His formerly wrinkled forehead relaxed easily, and his laughing rang out unreservedly. Resilience and serenity took the place of the restless nights and anxious days.

Encouraged by his improved feeling of self, Scott started investigating somatic exercises outside of his therapist's office. He made time for nature, danced freely, and practiced yoga; each of these experiences strengthened his bond with the outside world and himself.

Scott had experienced a deep sensation of aliveness a vigor that penetrated every part of his being—through somatic exercises that had also healed his previous scars. With his heart open and a fresh feeling of purpose, Scott welcomed life, free from the bonds of his trauma.

The Somatic Exercise Promise

John's tale is a moving reminder of how somatic exercises can help people recover their sense of self and heal trauma. Through a reconnection with the knowledge of the body, people like John can set out on a path of self-discovery and metamorphosis that leads to healing and completeness.

The pages that follow will go into the underlying ideas of somatic exercises, the complexities of the mind-body relationship, and offer useful tips and methods for integrating somatic activities into your everyday life. Somatic activities provide a route to recovery and development whether your goals are trauma, chronic pain, or just a greater connection to yourself.

Come along on this voyage of self-discovery and metamorphosis as we use somatic exercises to release the body and mind's healing potential.

Knowing Somatic Exercise

A wide variety of techniques geared at enhancing consciousness, healing, and integration of the mind-body connection are included in somatic exercise. Situated in the principles of somatic, a discipline that investigates the lived experience of the body, these exercises provide a comprehensive approach to health and wellbeing.

Fundamental to somatic training is the idea that the body has priceless knowledge and intelligence. By developing awareness of their own feelings, motions, and patterns, people can use this natural knowledge to promote recovery and development. Because somatic exercises emphasize interior awareness and self-discovery above physical fitness, they are potent instruments for personal change.

Inherent in somatic exercises is the idea of embodiment. Living in and giving one's body your whole attention in the here and now is known as embodiment. By means of somatic exercises including breath work, sensory awareness, and conscious movement, people are able to develop a closer relationship with their bodies, therefore promoting integration and wholeness.

Knowing the mind-body link is essential when doing somatic exercises. In contrast to Cartesian dualism, which holds that the mind and body are apart, somatic sees the mind and body as integral parts of one whole. This all-encompassing viewpoint recognizes how much psychological, emotional, and social aspects affect physical health and vice versa. Through somatic therapies that target the underlying source of physical complaints, people can noticeably enhance their general well-being.

There are several different modalities and approaches of somatic exercises, and each one provides special advantages and understanding of the mind-body link. Among the widespread somatic practices are:

Somatic Movement: The goal of these easy, exploratory exercises is to raise movement efficiency and awareness of body feelings. Slow and deliberate movement helps people to recognize and release tension points, which encourage rest and mobility.

Breathe work: A foundation of somatic exercises, conscious breathing methods assist people in controlling their nervous system, lowering tension, and developing presence. People can calm their nervous system and improve their general sense of well-being by noticing the depth and rhythm of their breath.

Body Scan: This mindfulness technique is methodically examining every part of the body, from head to toe, looking for any tension, pain, or relaxation. Greater ease and comfort in their bodies can be promoted by people recognizing and releasing areas of holding by becoming aware of their body sensations.

Sensory Awareness: To enhance the relationship between the body and mind, somatic exercises frequently include sensory awareness techniques. Those who are able to tune into the sights, sounds, scents, tastes, and textures of their surroundings can learn to be grounded and to stay in the present.

Emotional Release: Somatic exercises offer people a secure environment in which to investigate and communicate their feelings via movement and expression. Individuals can release trauma and pent-up energy held in the body, boosting emotional healing and resilience, by letting emotions flow unrestrictedly.

Somatic exercises, then, provide a comprehensive approach to health and well-being that recognizes the interdependence of the body and mind. People can use the transforming potential of somatic to heal old traumas, ease physical pain, and live more completely in the present moment by developing awareness, presence, and self-compassion.

Must Release Trauma

Millions of people worldwide suffer from trauma, ubiquitous and sometimes misdiagnosed phenomena. Trauma can have a significant and lasting impact on a person's physical, emotional, and psychological health whether it results from childhood maltreatment, combat experiences, natural disasters, or other causes of adversity. Trauma can become firmly embedded in the body without appropriate care, resulting in a wide range of medical symptoms, mental problems, and interpersonal problems.

Untreated trauma can have disastrous effects on people and society at large, so the need of trauma release cannot be emphasized. A person's capacity to flourish and find meaning and fulfillment is hampered by the impacts of trauma, which permeate every area of their life from addiction and relationship issues to chronic pain and sickness.

Through addressing the underlying reason of trauma stored in the body, somatic exercises provide a potent route to trauma release. While cognitive and verbal processing of traumatic events is the main focus of traditional talk therapy, somatic techniques address the bodily signs of trauma, such muscle tension, hyper vigilance, and dissociation. Somatic activities release buried trauma and restore a sense of completeness and well-being by using the body's natural ability for self-regulation and healing.

Somatic methods of trauma release are particularly advantageous since they get beyond the cognitive barriers that frequently develop in reaction to stressful events.

Somatic activities provide a kinder and more embodied way to healing than conventional talk therapy, which can occasionally re-traumatize people by making them revisit unpleasant experiences. Through attention to their own feelings and movements, people can access and release trauma stored in their bodies without feeling overburdened or re-traumatized.

To those healing from trauma, somatic activities also provide a sense of autonomy and empowerment. People actively take part in their own recovery process, learning to trust and listen to the knowledge of their bodies, rather than feeling like passive recipients of therapy. Regaining a feeling of control and autonomy over their lives, trauma survivors may find great empowerment in this sense of agency.

Somatic methods to trauma release also provide a comprehensive and integrative framework for healing that recognizes the interdependence of the mind, body, and spirit. Through physiologically addressing trauma, somatic exercises provide doors to more profound emotional and spiritual healing, enabling people to rediscover a deep sense of meaning and purpose in life and regain their sense of self.

In conclusion, it is impossible to exaggerate the value of trauma release, and somatic activities provide a potent and efficient way to deal with trauma that is stored in the body. Through mindfulness, present, and self-compassion cultivation, people can access the transforming potential of somatic to restore their natural ability for wholeness and well-being, heal old wounds, and ease physical pain.

PRINCIPLES OF SOMATIC WORKOUT

Somatic exercise refers to a wide range of techniques that aim to increase consciousness, facilitate healing, and promote the integration of the mind and body. Somatic exercises, based on the concepts of somatic, focus on the lived experience of the body. They provide a comprehensive approach to health and well-being that emphasizes inward awareness and self-discovery.

Somatic exercise refers to physical activities that involve conscious control and awareness of bodily movements, aiming to improve overall body function and movement efficiency.

Somatic exercise primarily entails engaging in any form of movement or practice that emphasizes the development of mindfulness towards bodily feelings, movements, and patterns. Contrary to conventional exercise methods that typically focus on exterior objectives like losing weight or building muscle, somatic exercises prioritize inward consciousness and self-control. By focusing on the immediate sensory experience of the body, individuals can access the inherent wisdom and intelligence that resides inside their own physical being.

Somatic exercises encompass a variety of forms, including gentle movements, breath work, mindfulness practices, and body awareness approaches. What unifies these different practices is their emphasis on the mind-body connection and their promise to facilitate healing and transformation at both the physical and emotional levels.

Principles of Somatic Workout

Embodiment: The core principle of somatic exercise is the idea of embodiment, which refers to fully experiencing and actively connecting with one's physical body in the present now. Rather than considering the body as a separate entity from the mind, somatic approaches highlight the interdependence of body and mind, emphasizing the significance of fostering awareness and present in the here and now.

Awareness: Somatic exercises prioritize the cultivation of awareness of bodily sensations, motions, and patterns. By paying attention to the various intricacies of bodily experience, individuals can gain a deeper understanding of themselves and their relationship to their bodies. This heightened awareness not only supports bodily well-being but also encourages emotional resilience and psychological growth.

Mindfulness: Mindfulness is a vital component of somatic exercise, helping individuals develops non-judgmental awareness of their thoughts, feelings, and body sensations. By bringing focused attention to their internal experience, individuals can become more attuned to the messages their bodies are sending them, allowing for increased self-regulation and stress reduction.

Integration: Somatic exercises aim to create integration of body, mind, and spirit, generating a sense of wholeness and well-being. Rather than compartmentalizing distinct components of the self, somatic techniques recognize the interconnectedness of all aspects of human experience, striving to achieve harmony and balance within the individual.

Empowerment: Somatic exercises allow individuals to take an active role in their own healing and growing process. By giving tools and procedures for self-exploration and self-regulation, somatic approaches enable individuals to tap into their own natural capacity for healing and transformation.

Gentleness and Non-Force: Unlike traditional forms of exercise that typically emphasize pushing through pain or discomfort, somatic exercises prioritize gentleness and non-force. By approaching movement with curiosity, openness, and compassion, individuals can create a safe and supportive atmosphere for discovery and healing.

Benefits of Somatic Exercises

Somatic exercises offer a plethora of benefits for persons wishing to improve their overall well-being and boost their quality of life. Rooted in the ideas of embodiment, awareness, and integration, these practices encourage healing and transformation at both the physical and emotional levels. Let's review some of the primary benefits of somatic exercises:

1. **Improved Body Awareness**: Somatic exercises assist individuals acquire a deeper awareness of their bodies, including sensations, movements, and patterns of tension. By tuning into their internal experience, individuals can become more attuned to the messages their bodies are sending them, allowing for improved self-regulation and self-care.

2. **Enhanced Relaxation and Stress Reduction**: Many somatic activities, such as deep breathing, gradual muscle relaxation, and gentle movement, enhance relaxation and stress reduction. By stimulating the body's relaxation response, these activities help individuals release tension trapped in the muscles and nervous system, resulting to a better sensation of peace and ease.

3. **Pain reduction and Management**: Somatic approaches to pain reduction focus on recognizing and releasing regions of tension and constriction in the body. By promoting greater ease of movement and alignment, these activities can decrease chronic pain and discomfort, helping patients restore their mobility and vitality.

4. **Improved Posture and Movement Efficiency**: Somatic exercises can assist individuals improve their posture and movement patterns, leading to better efficiency and ease of movement in daily activities. By releasing regions of tension and constriction, individuals can move more easily and naturally, minimizing the chance of injury and boosting general mobility.

5. **Emotional Regulation and Stress Resilience**: Somatic activities provide a safe and efficient technique of controlling emotions and processing painful experiences

stored in the body. By engaging in mindful movement and breath work, individuals can create space for emotional expression and release, encouraging increased resilience in the face of stress and hardship.

6. **Enhanced Body Image and Self-Confidence**: Through somatic exercises, individuals can develop a more positive body image and more self-confidence. By growing knowledge and acceptance of their bodies, individuals can transcend negative self-perceptions and embrace their intrinsic worth and beauty.

7. **Improved Sleep Quality**: Somatic activities can assist individuals enhance their sleep quality by increasing relaxation and stress reduction. By engaging in mild, relaxing routines before bedtime, individuals can prepare their bodies and brains for peaceful sleep, leading to better vigor and well-being.

8. **Increased awareness and Presence**: Somatic activities build awareness and presence by encouraging individuals to focus their attention on the present moment experience of their bodies. By tuning into their bodily sensations and motions, individuals can anchor themselves in the here and now, encouraging better clarity, attention, and inner calm.

9. **Promotion of Healing and Recovery**: Somatic exercises offer a holistic approach to healing and recovery, addressing the fundamental cause of physical and emotional imbalances stored in the body. By relieving tension, restoring mobility, and fostering relaxation, these activities assist the body's natural healing processes, leading to increased general well-being.

10. **Empowerment and Self-Care**: Somatic exercises allow individuals to take an active role in their own healing and well-being. By giving skills and techniques for self-exploration and self-regulation, these practices help individuals to tap into their own intrinsic capacity for healing and transformation, promoting a stronger sense of empowerment and self-care.

Safety Precautions and Considerations

While somatic exercises offer several benefits for persons looking to improve their general well-being, it's crucial to approach these activities with attention and care. Here are some safety measures and factors to keep in mind when partaking in somatic exercises:

- **Start slowly and progressively**: If you're new to somatic exercises, start slowly and progressively increase the intensity and duration of your practice over time. Listen to your body and follow its cues, stopping or changing exercises if you suffer any discomfort or pain.

- **Check a Healthcare practitioner**: If you have any underlying health disorders or concerns, it's crucial to check with a healthcare practitioner before commencing a somatic exercise program. They can provide assistance on relevant exercises and adaptations based on your unique needs and limits.

- **Respect Your Body's Limits**: It's crucial to respect your body's limits and avoid pushing yourself beyond your comfort zone. Somatic activities should feel soothing and nourishing, not harsh or forced. If you notice any discomfort or resistance, back off and consider different ways or alterations.

- **Stay Hydrated and Rested**: Proper hydration and rest are vital for supporting your body's natural healing processes and optimizing the effects of somatic workouts. Make sure to consume lots of water, get a proper amount of sleep, and emphasize self-care to promote your general well-being.

- **Avoid Overexertion**: While somatic exercises might be light and low-impact, it's still possible to overexert oneself if you're not careful. Pay attention to how your body responds to different workouts and alter your effort level accordingly. Remember that rest and recovery are just as vital as exercise and activity.

- **Listen to Your Body**: Your body is your best guide when it comes to somatic exercises. Pay attention to the feedback it delivers, including sensations, emotions, and energy levels. Trust your gut and alter your practice as needed to accommodate your body's specific requirements and preferences.

- **Adjust Exercises as Needed**: Don't be hesitant to adjust somatic exercises to suit your specific demands and talents. If a certain movement or posture feels painful or inaccessible, consider alternative variants or adaptations that feel more supportive and nutritious for your body.

- **Practice conscious Awareness**: Somatic activities are an opportunity to cultivate conscious awareness of your body and its sensations. Stay present and involved with your experience, observing any changes or insights that come during your practice. Mindful awareness can boost the advantages of somatic activities and deepen your connection to oneself.

- **Seek Professional advice**: If you're unclear about how to safely and effectively practice somatic exercises, consider receiving advice from a certified somatic therapist or instructor. They can provide specialized coaching, feedback, and support to help you get the most out of your practice while minimizing the risk of injury or discomfort.

The Body Connection

The mind-body connection is a fundamental aspect of human experience that has fascinated philosophers, scientists, and physicians for centuries. At its centre, this relationship refers to the intricate interplay between our thoughts, emotions, beliefs, and physical health. Understanding the mind-body connection is essential for unlocking the profound potential for healing and transformation that exists within each of us.

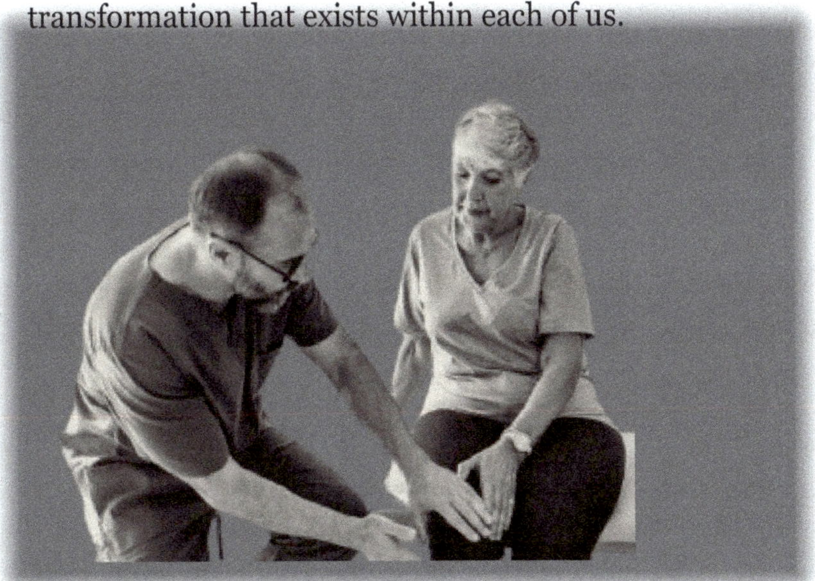

The Unity of Mind and Body

For much of history, Western medicine and philosophy regarded the mind and body as separate entities, operating independently of one another. This Cartesian dualism, as articulated by René Descartes in the 17th century, postulated a strict division between the realm of the mind (res cog tans) and the realm of the body (res extensor). However, emerging research in disciplines such as *psycho-neuron-immunology,* neurobiology, and somatic psychology has challenged this dualistic perspective, highlighting the interconnectedness of mind and body.

The Role of Emotions and Stress

Emotions play a central role in the mind-body connection, functioning as a bridge between our inner experiences and outward physiological responses. When we experience emotions such as pleasure, sadness, fear, or anger, our bodies respond in a variety of ways, releasing neurotransmitters, hormones, and other biochemical substances that influence our physiology.

Stress, in particular, can have profound effects on both mind and body. When we perceive a hazard or challenge, our bodies initiate the stress response, releasing hormones such as cortical and adrenaline to prepare us for action. While this response is essential for survival in acute situations, chronic stress can have detrimental effects on our health, contributing to a broad range of physical and psychological ailments.

Chronic stress has been linked to conditions such as cardiovascular disease, gastrointestinal disorders, immune dysfunction, and mental health disorders such as anxiety and depression. By comprehending the mind-body connection, we can learn to manage stress more effectively and promote greater well-being in our lives.

The Impact of Beliefs and Attitudes

Beliefs and attitudes also play a significant role in shaping the mind-body connection. Research has shown that our thoughts and beliefs can influence our physical health and well-being in profound ways. The placebo effect, for example, demonstrates the power of belief to produce measurable changes in physiology and health outcomes, even in the absence of active treatment.

Conversely, negative beliefs and attitudes can have detrimental effects on health and rehabilitation. The phenomenon known as the "nocebo effect" occurs when negative expectations or beliefs about a treatment or outcome contribute to worsened symptoms or outcomes. By cultivating positive beliefs and attitudes, individuals can employ the mind-body connection to promote healing and resilience.

Practical Applications

Understanding the mind-body connection has significant implications for health, healing, and personal growth. By cultivating awareness of our thoughts, emotions, and beliefs, we can learn to employ the power of the mind-body connection to promote greater well-being in our lives. Here are some practical applications of investigating the mind-body relationship:

- ***Mindfulness Practices***: Mindfulness practices such as meditation, yoga, and tai chi can help individuals cultivate greater awareness of their thoughts, emotions, and physiological sensations. By learning to observe and embrace these experiences without judgment, individuals can reduce stress, enhance self-regulation, and promote overall well-being.

- ***Stress Management Techniques***: Understanding the mind-body connection can help individuals develop effective stress management techniques to promote relaxation and resilience. Deep breathing exercises, progressive muscle relaxation, and guided imagery are just a few examples of techniques that can help individuals modulate their stress response and promote greater balance in their lives.

- ***Emotional Regulation Skills***: Emotion regulation skills are essential for navigating life's challenges and promoting emotional well-being. By learning to identify, express, and regulate their emotions in healthy ways, individuals can reduce the impact of stress on their bodies and minds and promote greater resilience in the face of adversity.

- ***Cognitive Restructuring***: Cognitive restructuring involves identifying and challenging negative beliefs and attitudes that contribute to stress and emotional distress. By replacing these beliefs with more positive and adaptive alternatives, individuals can promote greater well-being and cultivate a more optimistic outlook on life.

In summary, investigating the mind-body connection offers profound insights into the ways in which our thoughts, emotions, and beliefs influence our physical health and well-being. By cultivating awareness, practicing stress management techniques, and promoting emotional regulation skills, individuals can harness the power of the mind-body connection to promote greater resilience, vitality, and overall well-being.

The Neurophysiology of Trauma

Understanding the neurophysiology of trauma is critical for effectively treating its effects on the mind and body. Trauma, whether experienced as a single overwhelming incident or as repeated exposure to adversity, can have serious consequences for the brain, nervous system, and physiological functioning. Exploring the neurological basis of trauma can help us understand its consequences and design more tailored strategies for healing and recovery.

Stress Response and Brain

When confronted with a threat or danger, the body launches a complicated physiological reaction known as the stress response. The autonomic nervous system regulates this response, which includes the production of stress chemicals like cortical and adrenaline. In emergency situations, the stress response helps mobilize energy and resources to deal with the threat, allowing the individual to fight, run, or freeze in response to danger.

However, in the aftermath of traumatic experiences, the stress response may become deregulated, resulting in prolonged activation of the body's stress systems. Chronic activation can harm the brain, particularly areas like the amygdale, hippocampus, and prefrontal cortex.

- ***The Amygdale***: The amygdale is critical for emotional processing and memory formation. In response to a threat or danger, the amygdale becomes hyperactive, causing increased alertness and vigilance. This hyperactivity can exacerbate hyper arousal and hyper vigilance symptoms that are frequent in trauma patients.

- ***The Hippocampus***: The hippocampus plays a role in memory creation and consolidation, especially for contextual and episodic memories. Chronic stress and trauma have been linked to impaired hippocampus function, which leads to memory and learning deficiencies. This deficit can make it difficult to accurately recall distressing events and process them coherently.

- ***The Prefrontal Cortex***: The prefrontal cortex is important for executive tasks such as decision-making, impulse control, and mood regulation. Chronic stress and trauma can decrease prefrontal cortex function, making it difficult to regulate emotions and behavior. This impairment might show as symptoms such as impulsivity, emotional deregulation, and difficulties dealing with stressors.

The function of the autonomic nervous system

The autonomic nerve system (ANS) regulates many physiological functions, including heart rate, blood pressure, and digestion. It has two branches: the sympathetic nervous system (SNS), which controls the body's "fight or flight" reaction, and the parasympathetic nervous system (PNS), which promotes relaxation and restorative activities.

Trauma can cause the ANS to become deregulated, resulting in prolonged SNS activity and PNS suppression. This imbalance can lead to symptoms like hyper arousal, sleeplessness, and gastrointestinal problems. Understanding the involvement of the ANS in trauma allows us to develop therapies that restore balance and promote calm in the body.

The Effects of Trauma on Brain Structure and Function

Chronic trauma can have long-term impacts on brain structure and function, especially in areas involved in emotion regulation, memory processing, and stress response. Individuals who have experienced trauma have shown structural abnormalities such as changes in grey matter volume, white matter integrity, and petrochemical imbalance.

- ***Structural Changes***: Research has revealed that trauma can modify the structure of the brain, including changes in the size and connection of critical regions like the amygdale, hippocampus, and prefrontal cortex. These structural abnormalities may contribute to the issues in emotion control, memory processing, and stress response seen in trauma patients.

- ***Neurochemical Imbalances***: Trauma can disturb the brain's balance of neurotransmitters and hormones, resulting in deregulation of mood, arousal, and stress response. Neurotransmitter imbalances such as serotonin, dopamine, and nor epinephrine have been linked to the onset and persistence of trauma-related symptoms such as sadness, anxiety, and hyper arousal.

- ***Neuroplasticity***: Despite the devastating impacts of trauma on brain structure and function, the brain nevertheless has a remarkable capacity for neuroplasticity—the ability to reorganize and change in response to experience. This plasticity serves as a basis for healing and recovery, enabling people to build new coping mechanisms, learn adaptive behaviors, and restore nervous system equilibrium.

Somatic Exercises for Trauma Release

Somatic exercises provide a distinct and effective approach to trauma release by targeting the physiological manifestations of stress stored in the body. Unlike traditional types of therapy, which largely focus on cognitive and verbal processing of traumatic experiences, somatic techniques address the body's response to trauma, assisting clients in releasing tension, regulating arousal, and restoring nervous system balance.

How Somatic Exercises Help Trauma Release

- ***Nervous System Regulation***: Somatic exercises promote a transition from sympathetic dominance (fight or flight) to parasympathetic dominance (rest and relaxation). Gentle movements, breath work, and relaxation exercises can stimulate the body's relaxation response, lowering physiological arousal and fostering a sensation of safety and serenity.

- ***Release of Tension and Holding Patterns***: Trauma is commonly retained in the body as muscle tension, holding patterns, and somatic memories. Somatic exercises offer a safe and compassionate way to relieve these physical manifestations of trauma, helping people to unravel patterns of tension, release stored energy, and regain fluidity and ease of movement.

- ***Body-Mind Integration***: Somatic activities aid in the integration of body and mind, allowing people to reconnect with their embodied experiences and reclaim a sense of agency and sovereignty over their bodies. Individuals who cultivate awareness of physical sensations, movements, and limits can build better self-trust, self-compassion, and resilience in the face of trauma.

- ***Processing of Emotional Material***: Traumatic experiences are frequently retained in the body as unprocessed emotional material, resulting in symptoms such as flashbacks, nightmares, and disturbing thoughts. Somatic exercises offer a nonverbal method of processing and releasing emotions, allowing people to express and release pent-up energy and trauma stored in their bodies.

- ***Neuroplasticity Promotion***: Somatic activities, which involve conscious movement, sensory awareness, and breath work, enhance neuroplasticity—the brain's ability to reorganize and adapt to experience. Somatic activities promote resilience, flexibility, and adaptive responses to stress and adversity by forming new brain pathways and connections.

SOMATIC EXERCISE PREPARATIONS

Creating a safe and comfortable atmosphere is critical for engaging in somatic exercises effectively and reaping the maximum advantages. The atmosphere in which you practice has a significant impact on your capacity to relax, focus, and connect with your body. By creating a supportive environment, you may improve your somatic practice and encourage better ease and well-being. Here are some important considerations when building a secure and pleasant atmosphere for somatic exercises

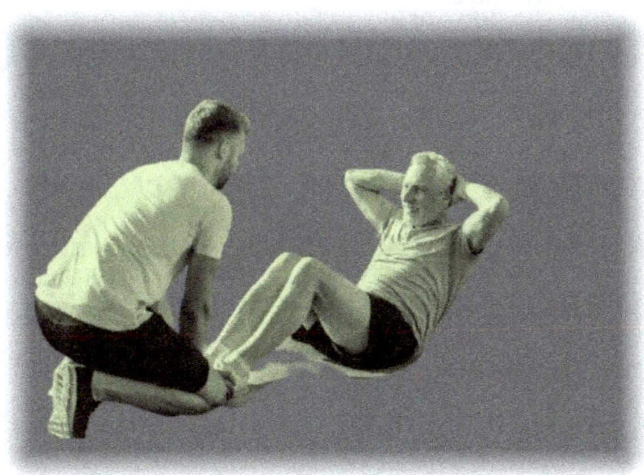

Providing a Safe and Comfortable Environment

- ***Select a Quiet and Private Space***: Find a quiet, private area where you may practice without interruptions or distractions. This could be a spare room, a section of your living room, or a private outdoor space. Reduce external distractions including noise, clutter, and visual stimuli to create a calm environment favorable to relaxation and introspection.

- ***Set the Mood***: Create a relaxing ambiance by dimming the lights, playing soothing music, or lighting candles or incense. Choose scents and sounds that will help you relax and feel more grounded and centered. Experiment with various sensory experiences to see what works best for you and helps your somatic practice.

- ***Use Comfortable Props and Support***: Collect whatever props or support you may require to make your practice more comfortable and pleasurable. Yoga mats, bolsters, blankets, cushions, and supportive pillows are all possible options. Arrange these props so that your body is supported and you can fully relax into each posture or exercise.

- ***Dress Comfortably***: Choose loose, comfortable clothing that allows for free mobility and breathing. Choose textiles that are smooth and soothing on your skin, and avoid anything that feels tight, confining, or restrictive. The goal is to achieve a state of ease and freedom in your body, allowing you to move and breathe organically.

- ***Ensure Adequate Ventilation***: Make sure the area is well-ventilated and at a comfortable temperature. Open the windows to bring in fresh air, or use a fan or air purifier to promote circulation. Proper ventilation can help you feel more alert, energized, and focused during your practice, which improves the whole experience.

- ***Clear Clutter and Create Space***: Remove any clutter or obstructions that may obstruct your movement or divert your focus. Create a sense of spaciousness and openness in the environment, so you may move freely and expansively without feeling constricted or confined. Arrange furniture and other items to encourage flow and ease of movement.

- ***Practice Mindful Awareness***: As you prepare for somatic practice, cultivate mindful awareness of your surroundings. Consider the feel of the floor beneath your feet, the texture of the props against your skin, and the quality of the light in the room. Pay close attention to how these sensory experiences affect your mood, energy levels, and overall sense of wellbeing.

- ***Personalize your room***: Make the room your own by adding personal touches that make you happy and comfortable. This could contain favorite artwork, photographs, or objects that have special importance to you. Surround yourself with positive reminders of your aims and goals for your somatic practice, and create a supportive environment that represents your individual preferences and personality.

- ***Set Intentions and Create Rituals***: Before starting your somatic practice, take a minute to set your intentions for the session and create any rituals or routines that will assist you shift into a state of presence and awareness. Lighting a candle, chanting a mantra or affirmation, or simply taking a few deep breaths can all help you centre yourself. Establishing these rituals might indicate to your body and mind that it is time to relax and become more receptive.

- ***Develop Self-Compassion and Acceptance***: Finally, approach your somatic practice with self-compassion and acceptance. Let go of any expectations or judgments about how your practice should appear or feel, and instead allow yourself to be present with whatever comes up. Trust that your body understands what it requires, and treat its wisdom with respect and care.

Mindfulness & Intention Setting

Warm-up Exercises

Warm-up activities are an important part of any somatic practice because they prepare the body and mind for movement, relaxation, and conscious awareness. Warm-up activities assist individuals in transitioning from the hectic pace of everyday life to a condition of present and readiness for somatic exploration by gradually awakening the body, releasing tension, and tuning into the breath. In this chapter, we'll look at a range of warm-up activities that induce relaxation, increase circulation, and improve body awareness in preparation for somatic practice.

Breath awareness

Begin by focusing on your breath, which serves as the anchor for mindfulness. Find a comfortable seated or sleeping posture, close your eyes if necessary, and take a few deep breathes in through the nose and out through the mouth. Consider the natural rhythm of your breathing, the rise and fall of your chest and abdomen, and the sensation of air entering and exiting your nostrils. Allow each breath to deepen and broaden your awareness, keeping you grounded in the present moment.

Gentle Stretching

Next, gradually stretch and awaken the body with easy movements that will relieve tension and promote flexibility. Begin with mild neck rolls, slowly rotating the head from side to side, followed by shoulder rolls, which include bringing the shoulders up towards the ears and rolling them back and down. Continue with arm circles, raising your arms high and circling them in both directions to expand up your chest and shoulders. Finally, stretch the spine by gradually arching and rounding the back while breathing to establish a comfortable range of motion.

Joint mobilization

Mobilize the body's key joints to improve circulation and range of motion. Begin with wrist circles, turning them in both directions to relieve tension in the hands and forearms. Next, perform ankle circles to loosen up the feet and lower legs. Continue doing knee raises, gently bringing one knee to the chest and then alternating sides to mobilize the hips and lower back. Finally, perform hip circles to loosen up the pelvis and alleviate tension in the lower body.

Centering and grounding

Take a moment to centre and ground yourself by connecting with the earth beneath you and the force of gravity. Stand with your feet hip width apart, knees slightly bent, and arms relaxed at your sides. Close your eyes and take a few deep breaths, feeling the soles of your feet firmly planted on the earth. Imagine a golden cord extending from the base of your spine to the soil, anchoring you in stability and strength. Allow yourself to feel supported and held by the earth, and use its nourishing energy to centre and anchor your body and mind.

Mindful Movement

Engage in mindful movement to awaken the body and develop present-moment awareness. Begin with slow, deliberate movements like gently rocking, swaying, or shaking to relieve stress and encourage the body's natural flow of energy. Move with fluidity and elegance, allowing each movement to emerge naturally from within, free of judgment or expectation. Pay close attention to the feelings in your body, the quality of your breath, and the subtle changes in your mood and energy as you move.

Body Scan

Finish your warm-up with a quick body scan, paying attention to each aspect of the body from head to toe. Begin at the crown of the head and carefully scan down the body, noting any places of tension, discomfort, or ease. Soften and relax into each sensation, letting any tension or holding dissipate with each breath. Bring a sense of curiosity and openness to your experience, and gently explore your body's environment.

Scene Five

CORE EXERCISES FOR TRAUMA RELIEF

Grounding practices are crucial tools for people looking to discharge trauma from their bodies and build a sense of safety, stability, and presence. Individuals can ground themselves in the present moment by connecting with the feelings of their bodies, laying the groundwork for healing and resilience. In this chapter, we'll look at three key grounding techniques: deep breathing, gradual muscle relaxation, and body scanning.

Grounding techniques

1. *Deep Breath*

Deep breathing, also known as diaphragmatic or belly breathing is an effective grounding technique for regulating the nervous system and promoting relaxation and serenity. Individuals can trigger the body's relaxation response and minimize the physiological arousal associated with trauma and stress by focusing on their breathing and activating their diaphragm.

To practice deep breathing:

- Take a comfortable seated or sleeping position, with one hand on your stomach and the other on your chest.

- If you're comfortable, close your eyes and take a few calm, deep breaths, breathing deeply through your nose and expelling completely through your mouth.

- As you breathe in, feel your belly inflate like a balloon, allowing your diaphragm to descend and fill your lungs with air.

- As you exhale, feel your belly gently compress, enabling the breath to entirely exit your body.

- Continue to breathe deeply and regularly, allowing each breath to increase your sensation of calm and presence.

Deep breathing can be done for a few minutes every day or whenever you need to ground yourself and relieve stress or worry.

2. *Progressive Muscle Relaxation*

Progressive muscle relaxation is a technique that involves gradually tensing and releasing various muscle groups in order to induce relaxation and reduce tension. Individuals who alternate between tension and relaxation can enhance their awareness of muscular tension and learn to release it voluntarily, promoting a sense of ease and comfort in the body.

To perform gradual muscular relaxation:

- Find a comfortable seated or sleeping posture, and close your eyes if necessary.

- Start by tensing the muscles in one portion of your body, such your fists or shoulders, and retaining the tension for a few seconds.

- Then, completely relieve the tension, allowing the muscles to relax and soften.

- Move on to the next muscle group, tensing and releasing tension as you work your way down the body from head to toe.

- Pay attention to the sensations of tension and relaxation in each muscle area, and note any changes in feeling between the two states.

- Continue to cycle through the muscle groups, allowing each wave of relaxation to enhance your sensation of peace and grounding.

Progressive muscle relaxation can be done alone or in conjunction with deep breathing to increase relaxation and stress reduction.

3: *Body Scanning*

Body scanning is a mindfulness practice that involves gradually bringing awareness to different regions of the body, from head to toe, and noting any sensations or feelings that arise in each location. Individuals can anchor themselves in the present moment by focusing on their physical sensations and cultivating a sense of embodied awareness and presence.

To perform body scanning:

- Find a comfortable seated or sleeping posture, and close your eyes if necessary.

- Start by paying attention to the sensations in your feet, noting any feelings of warmth, tingling, or pressure.

- Move your focus slowly up your body, inspecting each place in turn, starting with your legs and ending with your head.

- Observe any regions of tension, discomfort, or ease without criticizing or attempting to change them.

- Allow your attention to rest on each sensation for a few moments before moving on to the next, building curiosity and openness to your surroundings.

- Once you've scanned your entire body, take a few deep breaths and allow yourself to completely relax into the present now.

Body scanning can be done as a single exercise or as part of a regular mindfulness regimen to enhance relaxation, self-awareness, and grounding.

In conclusion, grounding techniques like as deep breathing, progressive muscle relaxation, and body scanning are useful tools for those looking to release trauma held in their bodies and build a sense of safety, stability, and present. Individuals who include these practices into their daily routine can improve their relationship with their body, regulate their nervous system, and encourage greater resilience and well-being in the face of hardship.

Stress and tension release

Three potent somatic exercises meant to release tension and stress held in the body will be covered in this part. Through their promotion of relaxation, body awareness, and nervous system restoration, these exercises assist people in releasing the physical effects of trauma and developing a sense of ease and well-being.

Movements of the Somatic Body

Gentle, flowing movement patterns called somatic movement flows are intended to help the body relax, increase mobility, and release tension. Through a sequence of integrated movements performed slowly and deliberately, people can improve body awareness, increase circulation, and release patterns of muscular holding, therefore promoting a sense of embodied presence and vitality.

Practice somatic movement flows

Start by adjusting to a comfortable standing position with knees slightly bent and feet hip-width apart.

In - Spend a few minutes focusing and relating to your breath, letting your awareness to become anchored in your body.

- Waken the body and pay attention to your physical feelings, begin with a basic warm-up exercise like soft rocking or swaying from side to side.

- Start by gradually experimenting with a variety of fluid motions that let your body move naturally and instinctively in reaction to your breath and the sensations inside of it.

- With mindfulness and curiosity, move, noticing the quality of each step and any tightness or limitations you may come across.

- Play about with various movement patterns, such reaching, twisting, bending, and flowing, to let your body speak for itself naturally and spontaneously.

- Maintaining your own pace, investigate the whole range of movements at your disposal, and note any changes in your energy, attitude, or bodily sensations as you go.

- Several minutes of movement later, progressively end your practice, giving yourself an opportunity to relax and note how your body and mind are feeling.

- Regular practice of somatic movement flows can improve body awareness, relaxation, and mobility either alone or as part of a wider somatic practice.

Exercises for Disposal of the Pelvic Floor

Through the release of tension and tightness in the pelvic floor muscles, the pelvic floor release exercises encourage relaxation, circulation, and vitality in the pelvic area. Because the pelvic floor supports the pelvic organs, keeps bladder and bowel control, and promotes sexual function, any imbalances or limits in this area must be addressed.

To do movements for the release of the pelvic floor,

- Start by settling into a cozy sitting or sleeping posture with your spine straight and your feet flat on the floor.
- Breathe deeply a few times, letting each exhale soften and relax your body.
- At the base of your pelvis, between your pubic bone and tailbone, are the pelvic floor muscles. - Bring them to your attention.

- As if you were squeezing and pushing the muscles inside and upward, contract and release these muscles gradually.
- Maintaining a rhythmic contraction and relaxation of the pelvic floor muscles, match your breathing to the actions.
- Gently tense and raise the pelvic floor muscles as you exhale, bringing them up towards your navel.
- Release the contraction as you inhale, letting the muscles of the pelvic floor totally relax and soften.
- As you grow more at ease with the practice, progressively lengthen and intensify the contractions as you repeat this pattern of contraction and release for a number of breaths.
- Prevent overstretching or strain, take breaks as needed and pay attention to your body's signals.

Exercises for the pelvic floor release can help people decompress, enhance pelvic floor function, and increase awareness of and connection to this important body part.

Techniques for Release of the Shoulder and Neck

Techniques for shoulder and neck release aim to reduce tension and stiffness in the muscles of the shoulders, neck, and upper back, therefore encouraging ease of movement, relaxation, and mobility in these areas. Particularly in those who have gone through trauma or who spend extended periods of time seated at a desk or computer, the shoulders and neck are typical locations of tension and stress buildup.

To work on neck and shoulder releases

Start by assuming a comfortable sitting or standing position with your shoulders back and your spine straight.

- o Breathe deeply a couple times, letting each exhale cause your body to soften and relax.
- Bringing your attention to your shoulders, note any knots or pain there.
- Allowing your shoulder blades to slide down your back, gently move your shoulders up towards your ears on an inhale and back and down on an exhale.
- Many repetitions of this exercise should be made, letting your breath dictate the beat and flow of the action.

- Feel the stretch along the side of your neck as you next slowly tilt your head to one side, bringing your ear towards your shoulder, and hold for a few breaths.
- Holding for a few breaths, tilt your head to the other side and repeat from centre.
- Stretching your neck and shoulders and investigating any places of tightness or restriction you may come across, keep moving deliberately.
- In order to prevent strain or pain, take your time and pay attention to your body's input as you modify the length and intensity of each stretch.

Through the release of tension, improvement of posture, and reduction of stiffness and discomfort in the upper body, shoulder and neck release techniques can enable people move more easily and freely of their bodies.

In conclusion, people who wish to create a sense of relaxation, mobility, and well-being as well as release trauma held in the body can benefit much from the somatic exercises for releasing tension and stress. Through the daily practice of somatic movement flows, pelvic floor release exercises, and shoulder and neck release techniques, people may encourage increased awareness, ease, and resilience in their bodies and minds, therefore promoting a deeper sense of connection and vitality in their lives.

Enhancing Body Sensation and Awareness

Three transforming techniques meant to improve bodily awareness and sensation will be examined in this part. These practices are meant to help us feel more embodied presence and energy, to strengthen our relationship with the body, and to raise awareness of physical sensations. Deeper awareness of our bodily experience helps us to more skillfully negotiate the complexity of trauma with more fortitude, empathy, and insight.

Exercising the Body Mapping

Exercises in body mapping are effective means of raising consciousness of the structure, function, and interconnection of the body. Through investigation of the anatomical landmarks, movement patterns, and regions of tension or restriction in the body, people can get a deeper knowledge of their physical selves and a closer bond with them.

To work through body mapping exercises

Start by getting into a relaxed, tall-spin seated or standing stance.

- Breathe deeply a few times, letting your attention to drop into your body and the here and now.
- Moving progressively upward through your legs, pelvis, belly, chest, arms, hands, neck, and head, begin with your feet and focus on each area of your body.
- Look for any sensations, such warmth, tingling, pressure, or pain, in every part of your body.
- Gently examine each region with your hands, following the lines of your body and noting any places where you feel tight, tense, or constrained.
- Watch how you move and note any places where you might feel resistance or stiffness.
- Spend some time and go slowly through every area of your body so that you may completely feel and live in each moment.
- Take a few minutes after finishing your body mapping exercise to consider your experience and any new discoveries or observations that came to you.

- Exercises in body mapping can help people become more appreciative of their bodies, more conscious of their sensations, and more integrated and entire in their physical experience.

Techniques for Sensory Awareness

Techniques for sensory awareness aim to raise consciousness of touch, temperature, pressure, and proprioception—among other sensory experiences of the body. People can strengthen their relationship with their bodies and develop a more embodied presence and awareness by focusing on the rich tapestry of sensory information that is accessible to us at any one time.

To work on methods of sensory awareness

- Take up a cozy sitting or sleeping position and close your eyes to let your body unwind.
- Breathe deeply a few times, letting your awareness spread throughout your whole body.

- Start by drawing attention to the many sensory sensations that your body offers, beginning with touch.

- Take note of how your clothing feels on your skin, how the ground feels underfoot, and where in your body you feel warm or cool.

- Explore further sensory sensations, such the rhythm of your heartbeat, the feeling of your breath coming in and out of your body, and the minute changes in your posture and movement.

- Identify any tightness or pain in your body, then openly and curiously investigate these feelings.

- Let yourself to completely experience every sense, letting whatever comes to mind to be there in your consciousness without any expectations or criticism.

- After finishing your sensory awareness exercise, pause to consider your experience and any new discoveries or observations that came to you.

Techniques for sensory awareness can help people become more aware of their body sensations, appreciate the richness of their sensory experience more deeply, and feel more anchored and present in their physical experience.

Practices for Somatic Experiencing

Based in somatic psychology, somatic experience techniques seek to help the body's nerve system release trauma that has been held there. People who progressively reduce patterns of tension and reactivity can promote healing and resilience in the face of adversity by gently examining feelings, emotions, and bodily reactions linked to trauma.

Practices for somatic experiencing

- Take up a cozy sitting or sleeping position and close your eyes to let your body unwind.
- Take a few long breaths and let your awareness to spread across your whole body.
- Start observing, judgment- and analysis-free, any feelings, feelings, or physical reactions that come to mind.
- Find any places in your body where you feel tight, uncomfortable, or activated, and gently and compassionately investigate these feelings.
- Your body will direct the release and integration process if you let yourself to move and express

whatever impulses or motions that come to you naturally.

- Allow whatever comes up to be kindly and acceptingly acknowledged and observed as you allow the wisdom of your body to lead you through the somatic experience.

- Following your somatic experiencing practice, give yourself a few minutes to relax and process your experience so that you can come back to calm and focused state.

In addition to facilitating integration and healing, somatic experiencing techniques can help people develop a feeling of wholeness and resilience in their physical and emotional experiences.

To sum up, those who want to improve their body awareness and sensation will benefit much from the body mapping exercises, sensory awareness approaches, and somatic experience practices. Through enhancing our relationship with our body, raising consciousness of our physical sensations, and

Scene Six

ADVANCED SOMATIC STRATEGIES

Here we explore sophisticated somatic techniques meant to enhance the bodily experience, promote emotional release, and promote integration and connection both with oneself and with others. These practices are intended for people who are prepared to investigate more sophisticated methods for healing and transformation and who have already gained a basic understanding of somatic work.

Movement and Breath work Integration

A potent somatic exercise, breath work and movement integration blends deliberate movement with the rhythmic flow of the breath to produce energetic balance, profound relaxation, and tension release. Breathing and moving in time allows people to build present, reach higher levels of embodied awareness, and utilize the body's natural knowledge and energy.

Practice: Movement with the Breath

- Start in a relaxed, tall spined seated or standing position.
- Closing your eyes and taking a few long breaths, let your consciousness to come into contact with your body and the here and now.
- Begin by moving your body naturally and intuitively, letting your breath direct the rhythm and flow of your actions.
- With your arms and chest stretching upward and outward as you inhale, open and expand your body.
- Breathe-guide the movement as you exhale, contract and release, pulling your arms and torso inward and lower.
- Keep breathing while moving, experimenting with several rhythms and patterns to express and release any holding or tension in your body.
- Let the movement to naturally end, then pause for a short while to recover and process what you've experienced.

Benefits

- It raises sensitivity and physical awareness.
- Encourages unwinding and lowering of tension.
- Enables flow and alignment of the energy.
- It increases awareness and presence.

Emotional Release Techniques Exploration

Investigating emotional release techniques entails providing a secure and encouraging environment in which people may express and work through bodily stored feelings. People who practice somatic techniques that promote the discharge of emotional energy can break free from avoidance and repression tendencies and advance towards more emotional freedom, authenticity, and wholeness.

Emotional Catharsis Practice

1. Locate a quiet, private area and a comfortable sitting or reclining position.

2. Closing your eyes and taking a few long breaths, let your consciousness to come into contact with your body and the here and now.

3. Think back on any sentiments you have been concealing or clinging to.

4. Let yourself feel, hear, or gesture your way through these feelings completely, without restriction or criticism.

5. Give yourself permission to express whatever comes to you spontaneously so that the emotions' energy may pass through you and leave your body.

6. As you work through the exercise, take note of any thoughts, feelings, or insights that come to you. This will help you to completely witness and respect your experience.

7. After several minutes of emotional catharsis, progressively end the exercise by inhaling deeply, relaxing, and assimilating your experience.

Benefits

- o   Let's go of bottled up emotional energy in the body.
- o   Advances integration and healing of the emotions.
- o   Boosts own expression and awareness.
- •   It fosters genuineness and emotional resiliency.

Exercises in Somatic with Partners and Groups

Engaging with others to enhance the somatic experience, build connection, and support and heal one another is the essence of partner and group somatic exercises. Sharing the somatic journey with others allows people to benefit from the group's collective knowledge and energy as well as to feel a feeling of community, empathy, and belonging.

Mirror Movement Practice

- Standing facing each other at a comfortable distance, pair up with a partner.
- Spend a short while focusing on your spouse and feeling their energy.
- Start reflecting one other's motions, leading and following in turns and letting the motions come to you naturally and instinctively.
- As you practice, pay attention to any feelings that come up and let yourself to completely experience the shared movement and sense of connection.
- After a few minutes of mirror movement, progressively wind up the exercise, giving your partner a few minutes to thank you and think back on your experience.

Benefits

- o Promotes human connection and empathy.
- • Encourages healing and support amongst oneself.
- • Increases awareness of nonverbal and communication.
- • Supports a feeling of community and belonging.

All things considered, the sophisticated somatic approaches of combining movement and breath work, investigating emotional release methods, and participating in partner and group somatic exercises provide potent avenues for enhancing the somatic experience, promoting healing and transformation, and promoting integration and connection both with oneself and with others. By including these techniques into their somatic work, people can reach deeper levels of consciousness, let go of stress and emotion, and access the great wisdom and vigour of the body-mind system.

Scene Seven

ACCOMMODATING SOMATIC EXERCISES TO PARTICULAR TRAUMA

We investigate in this part how somatic exercises can be customized to deal with certain kinds of trauma, giving people focused methods for resilience and healing. Knowing the particular difficulties and ways that various traumas present themselves allows people to tailor their somatic practice to their own requirements and further their own healing and well-being.

Complex Trauma and PTSD

Trauma from overwhelming or traumatic events, such combat, childhood abuse, or interpersonal violence, can manifest as either Complex Trauma or Post-Traumatic Stress Disorder (PTSD). Both the body and the mind may be profoundly affected by these events, resulting in symptoms including emotional deregulation, intrusive thoughts, hyper vigilance, and flashbacks. Specific somatic exercises designed to treat PTSD and Complex Trauma concentrate on nervous system regulation, safety and grounding promotion, and the release and integration of painful memories and feelings.

Grounding Techniques Practice

- Start by locating a comfortable sitting or standing posture and centering and re-connecting with your body with a few deep breaths.
- Using your senses to anchor yourself in the present, bring your attention to your surrounds. Take on the noises, sights, and sensations of your feet on the floor.
- To stay in the present, use grounding techniques include tactile stimulation, visualization, or rhythmic movement. Imagine, for instance, that you are a tree, or tap your thighs lightly to get a rhythmic feeling.
- To provide a sense of security and stability and to assist regulate your nervous system, practice grounding techniques often, particularly during periods of increased stress or worry.

Features

- The nervous system is helped to regulate.
- It stimulates stability and safety.
- Lessens dissociative and hyper vigilance symptoms.

Anxiety and Panic Disorders

Persistent sensations of anxiety, worry, or dread are hallmarks of anxiety and panic disorders; they are frequently accompanied by physical symptoms such a fast heartbeat, perspiration, shaking, and short of breath. The goals of somatic exercises designed to treat anxiety and panic disorders are to promote relaxation and self-soothing abilities, quiet the nervous system, and reduce the body's stress reaction.

Deep Breathing Exercises Practices

- Whether seated or reclining comfortably, choose a place to close your eyes.
- Count to four while you take a long, steady breath in through your nose.
- After holding your breath for a while, softly exhale through your mouth, counting to six as you do so.

- Carry on breathing this manner, paying attention to the duration and pattern of your breath and letting each exhale be slower and longer than the inhalation.
- As you take each breath, notice how peace and relaxation permeate your body, and let yourself to give yourself over to the present.
- To help relax and build a sense of calm and well-being, do calming breathing exercises often, particularly during periods of increased anxiety or panic.

Benefits

- Lowers physiological excitement and calms the nervous system.
- It encourages rest and lessens panic and anxiety symptoms.
- It enhances abilities in self-control and self-awareness.

Somatization and Dissociation

Dissociation and somatization are coping strategies for handling stressful or overwhelming events in which one separates from their ideas, feelings, or physical sensations. Aiming to promote grounding and embodiment, integration and connection with oneself and the present moment, and increased awareness of body sensations, somatic exercises designed to alleviate dissociation and somatization.

Body Scan Meditation Practice

1. To centre and unwind your body, find a comfortable sitting or sleeping posture and take a few deep breaths.

2. Focus on your breathing and let it to lead you into a calm and present state.

3. Beginning with your feet, slowly move over every section of your body, noting any sensations or emotions in each place.

4. Observe any places of tightness, pain, or numbness, and let yourself to compassionately and curiously investigate these feelings.

5. Let warmth and ease to permeate your body with every breath, relaxing and releasing any places of holding or resistance.

6. Keep moving your body from your feet to your head, letting yourself completely live and experience every moment.

7. Take some time to relax and process your experience after finishing the body scan so that you can get back to being composed and at ease.

Benefits

- Sharpens perception of physical sensations.
- It encourages embodiment and grounding.
- It helps one become more integrated and connected to the here and now.

In conclusion, customizing somatic techniques to successfully address the particular difficulties and manifestations of each kind of trauma is the key to personalizing somatic exercises to certain trauma types. People can foster recovery and resilience as well as a higher sense of well-being and connection in their life by including grounding exercises, soothing breathing exercises, body scan meditations, and other focused somatic exercises into their practice.

UPHOLDING PROGRESS AND ROUTINES

Here we look at ways to keep making progress and include somatic activities into everyday life as a kind of self-care. Through knowledge of the long-term advantages of somatic exercise, journaling and introspection, and including somatic activities into everyday routines, people can maintain their progress, encourage continuous healing, and develop a stronger sense of resilience and well-being.

Long-Term Advantages of Somatic Exercise

Long-term effects of somatic workouts go well beyond the momentary alleviation of symptoms. People can have significant changes in their physical, emotional, and psychological well-being over time by consistent somatic practice.

- ***Benefits to the Body:***
  Exercises of the somatic kind ease tension in the muscles enhance flexibility and posture. Frequent

practice can lead to increased body awareness and resilience, which in turn improves balance, coordination, and general physical health.

- ***Affects Emotionally***

  Somatic exercises offer people a secure and encouraging environment in which to investigate and work through emotions held in the body. Increased emotional fortitude, self-awareness, and better mood control can all result from this over time.

- ***Advantages for Psychologists***

  People that do somatic exercises get better at self-regulating and finding coping strategies for stress and hardship. Mindfulness and presence training can help people feel more empowered and in control of their lives as well as lessen the symptoms of anxiety, sadness, and trauma-related illnesses.

Journaling and Self-Reflection

Journaling and introspection are useful instruments for expanding the somatic experience and obtaining understanding of one's ideas, emotions, and physical experiences. Through consistent introspection on their somatic practice and journaling of their experiences, people can monitor their development, spot trends and triggers, and develop more self-awareness and self-understanding.

Somatic Journaling Practice

1. Take a moment each day to consider your somatic practice and your bodily experiences.

2. Start by recording whatever bodily and mental sensations, emotions, or ideas you have before, during, and after your somatic practice.

3. Consider any revelations or observations—such as points of tension or release, emotions that erupted, or breathing or movement patterns—that came to you during your exercise.

4. Think about how your somatic practice affects your relationships, career, or general feeling of wellbeing.

5. Ask yourself questions in your notebook, such "What am I feeling in my body right now?" or "What patterns or themes are emerging in my somatic practice?"

6. Write anything comes to mind and convey it on the page. Write without restriction.

Making Daily Practices Somatic

Maintaining progress and encouraging continuous healing and well-being need including somatic techniques into daily life. People can develop more presence, mindfulness, and connection with themselves and the outside world by including somatic exercises into their everyday routines and activities.

Mindful Movement Pauses

- Move deliberately and perform somatic exercises during little breaks during the day.
- Include easy exercises like body scans, deep breathing, and stretching into your regular schedule—for example, right before bed or after lunch.
- Turn commonplace activities—like walking slowly, washing dishes with mindfulness, or sitting in meditation while standing in line—into chances for somatic practice.
- Use your body's feelings while you move and go about your everyday business as anchors for your awareness in the here and now.
- Observe how including somatic activities into your everyday routine affects your general level of energy,

well-being, and capacity to handle stress and obstacles.

To sum up, keeping up with progress and self-care routines includes realizing the long-term advantages of somatic exercise, reflecting and journaling, and incorporating somatic activities into everyday life. People can maintain their development, encourage continuous healing, and develop a stronger sense of resilience and well-being in their life by developing a regular somatic practice and a deeper relationship with themselves.

CONCLUSSION

The main ideas covered in this book are summed up in this last section, along with encouragement for ongoing practice and some last comments on somatic healing for trauma release.

Key Concepts Recap

We have covered the transforming potential of somatic exercises for trauma release throughout this book. We have studied the neurophysiology of trauma, the mind-body connection, and the foundations of somatic exercise—breathing exercises, movement exercises, and grounding techniques. We have developed somatic exercises to address certain traumas, such PTSD, anxiety, and dissociation, and we have talked about sophisticated techniques for intensifying the bodily experience and encouraging continuous recovery. We have underlined throughout the somatic journey the value of safety, self-awareness, and self-care, and we have included materials and additional reading for anybody who want to learn more about and practice somatic exercises.

Encouragement for Ongoing Practice

We invite you to approach your practice as you proceed on your somatic journey with openness, compassion, and curiosity. Recall that the body stores layers of trauma, and healing is a process that requires time and patience to untangle. As you experiment with various techniques and experiences, be kind to yourself and believe that your body will know best how to lead you towards completeness and recovery. Please know that you are not travelling alone; a large network of people and resources is at your disposal to help you at every stage. Maintain your relationships with both yourself and other people, and never be afraid to ask for help when you need it.

Final Thoughts on Trauma Release via Somatic Healing

We would want to thank you very much for starting this somatic healing path for trauma release in closing. May you keep developing presence, fortitude, and compassion in your life and may the wisdom of your body bring you comfort and release. May you find fresh levels of joy, empowerment, and healing as you include somatic activities into your everyday life, and may your bravery and dedication to living fully and truly motivate others.

Recall that recovery is a lifetime path of self-discovery and change rather than a destination. With courage and an open heart, may you welcome this trip and discover beauty and grace at every turn.

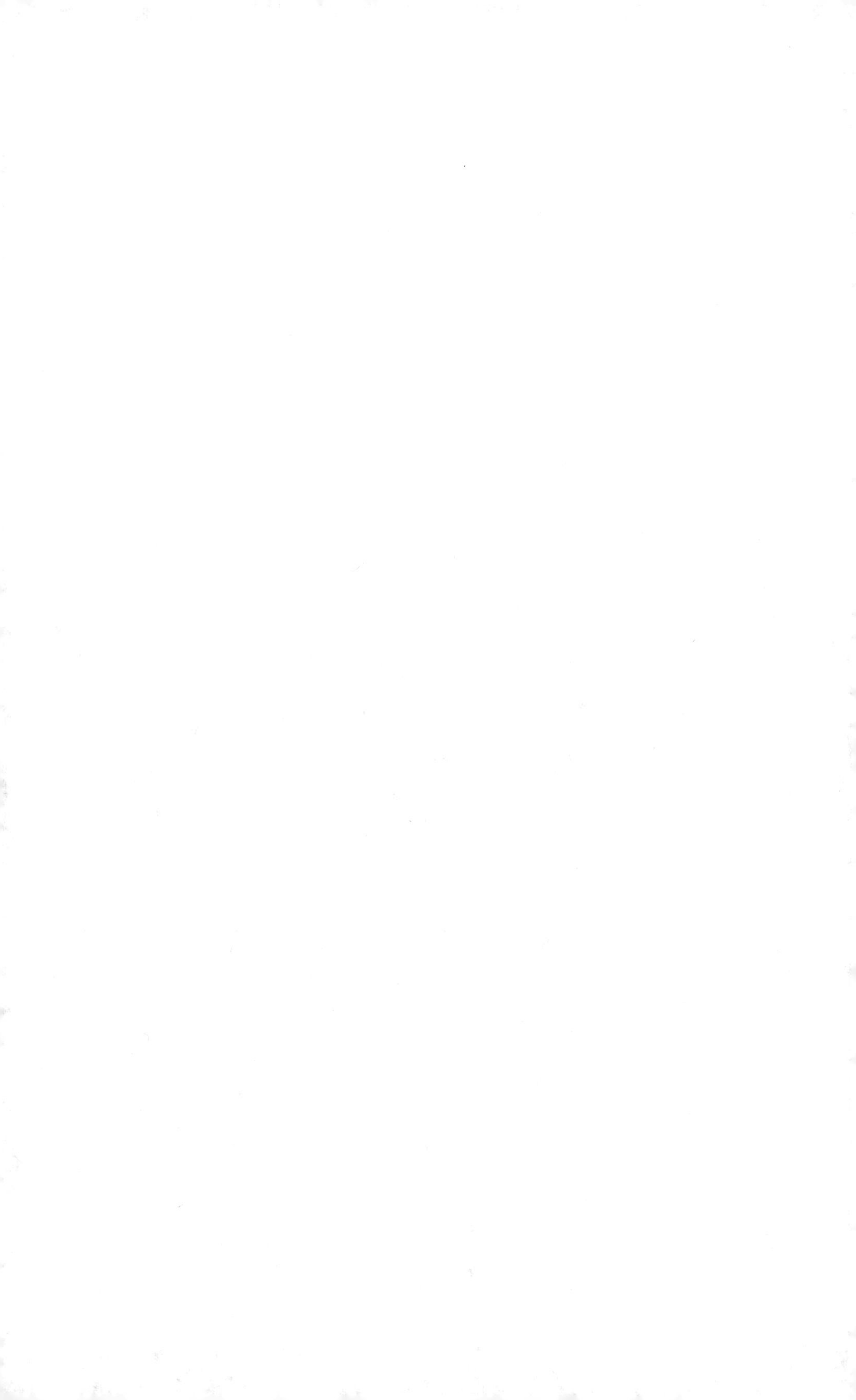